COMPUTER EYE STRESS

HOW TO AVOID IT, HOW TO ALLEVIATE IT

- Exercises to strengthen eyes for greater comfort and productivity during prolonged computer work
- Why your computer may be straining your eyes
- How to adjust your work environment to ease eye fatigue

Dr. R. ANTHONY HUTCHINSON

Computer Eye-Stress

Computer Eye-Stress

How to Avoid It;
How to Alleviate It

Dr. R. Anthony Hutchinson

M. Evans and Company, Inc.
New York

Library of Congress Cataloging in Publication Data

Hutchinson, R. Anthony.
  Computer eye-stress.

  1. Eyestrain. 2. Video display terminals—Hygienic
aspects. I. Title.
RE48.H87 1985   617.7   85-1476

ISBN 0-87131-457-6 (pbk.)

M. Evans and Company, Inc.
216 East 49 Street
New York, New York 10017

Interior Design by Michael Kelly, The Word Shop, San Diego
Illustrations by Ed Roxburgh, The Word Shop, San Diego

Manufactured in the United States of America

9 8 7 6 5 4 3 2 1

Acknowledgements

I would like to acknowledge the assistance of several people: Alan Davidson, Ph.D., Bernard Press, O.D., Randall Yumori, O.D., and David Workman all gave me excellent advice on both the content of the book and my writing style. Pat Powell and Pat Bochstahler helped with manuscript preparation. Finally, I would like to thank Mary Jo Crowley for ensuring that the right person read the manuscript.

for mom and dad

Contents

Introduction

It wasn't very long ago that I realized computers are everywhere! I've always been something of a computer aficionado; over the years I've taken quite a few computer courses and once even built what's called an "analogue computer." I've always enjoyed working with computers, but I enjoy working with people even more. That's why my career path led me to become an optometrist instead of a computer engineer. I did marry a computer engineer (although not for that reason). Maybe because of my lack of professional involvement with the computer world, I hadn't really noticed how much and how quickly that world was expanding.

Then I became aware of that vast growth through my practice as an optometrist. In the last few years, an increasing number of my patients have been complaining of computer-related eyestrain. The most common ailments have been headaches, blurry vision (both distant and close-up), itching and burning eyes, double vision, and a major dose of general eye fatigue (Figure 1).

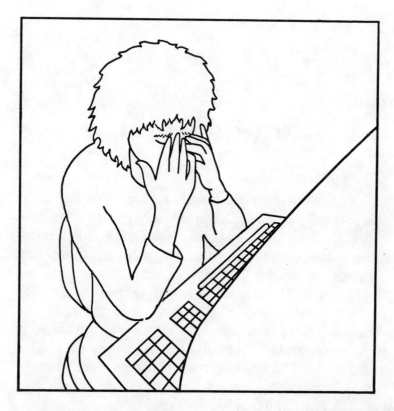

Figure 1. More than 75 percent of computer users report some form of visual discomfort related to the use of VDT terminals.

It wasn't the computer itself that was causing these problems, but rather the **video display terminal** (called the VDT, computer screen, or computer monitor). VDTs can be found anywhere and everywhere – in video arcades, newsrooms, airport terminals, and nearly one-tenth of the homes in America! And they've literally taken over the office environment, from mailroom cubbyholes to presidential suites.

The symptoms I describe here are collectively known as **VDT fatigue**. How to combat VDT fatigue is what this book is all about.

Increasing Problems

Computers and VDTs have been around for a while, but VDT fatigue is only beginning to surface in public awareness. Why? The handful of "early" scientists and engineers who worked with VDTs were strongly motivated individuals in a fascinating new field of "high technology." They considered their visual discomforts to be mere occupational hazards, work-related stress factors they had to endure as they incessantly produced bigger and better computer systems. It wasn't anything, they supposed, that two weeks in the sun wouldn't cure.

But now that so many of the rest of us are working with computers – most of us for the first time – the complaints of VDT eye-stress are becoming a major threat to productivity and user safety. Over 75 percent of computer users report some form of visual discomfort while using a terminal. And, as more and more of us spend more and more time at the VDT, the problem is steadily worsening. It's estimated that by 1990, 50 percent of American workers will use computer terminals, some 40 million homes will be equipped with them, and computers will be as common in schools as chalkboards are now!

Solving Problems

My purpose in this book is to help *you* to be as comfortable and safe as possible while working at your computer terminal. I want you to know the causes (and cures) of eyestrain and visual discomfort. Improper lighting, glare, and reflection are all part of the problem, as are flickering screens, color, screen brightness, and letter size. I'll talk about the best design for a comfortable work station – chair height, screen distance (from your eyes), and so on. I also want to address special visual problems, such as nearsightedness and farsightedness, weak eye muscles, and the hazards children face when they work with VDTs. Computers may give our children genius status by the age of twelve, but let's make sure they don't cause them eye damage en route!

The two-part plan at the end of this book gives easy-to-follow steps for reducing and preventing VDT fatigue, as well as easing discomfort caused by video terminals. Like most remedies, these won't work by themselves; but with a little understanding and patience on your part, you can make *your* computer eye-stress a thing of the past!

What Is a VDT?

A VDT (video display terminal) is a cathode ray tube, very much like a television set, which has been specially designed for use with computers (Figure 2). In a cathode ray tube (CRT), a beam of electrons is shot from the back of the tube to the screen at the front. This beam scans across the display screen in horizontal lines. The back of the screen has been coated with a chemical phosphor. The phosphor screen glows whenever the electron beam strikes it. As the electron beam scans back and forth, it illuminates the **raster structure**, those tiny dots that compose each character that appears on the screen.

Your television works the same way. However,

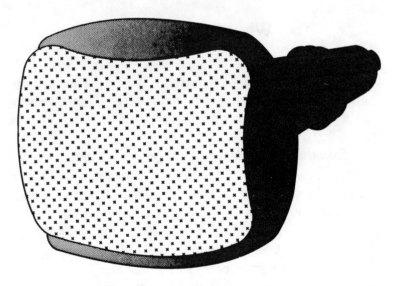

Figure 2. A VDT is a specially designed cathode ray tube (CRT). Although VDTs are similar to the CRTs used in televisions, a slower-fading phosphor makes them easier on the eyes.

there are a number of differences between a television set and a VDT, and good reasons for doing VDT work on a VDT (and not on a TV set). A television picture is usually a moving image. The phosphor fades quickly so that one image can merge smoothly into the next. But when a quick-fade phosphor is used to show relatively steady images (such as raster-structured characters), you'll find a high incidence of screen "flicker." Flicker can drive your eyes crazy. VDTs have a slower-fading phosphor, and hence a less apparent flicker. Generally, a VDT is far better for computer work than a television set attached to a computer.

What Is Eyestrain?

If you use a VDT frequently, I'll bet you already know the symptoms of eyestrain. Your eyes burn; your head pounds; the images on your screen lose focus or "double up." But what's really happening to your eyes to cause the eyestrain?

Eyestrain can be brought on in several different ways. The muscles that control eye movement can become tired. Or the focusing muscles can tire. Or your brain can have so much difficulty trying to decipher what you're looking at that both your eyes *and* your brain can tire out. (Have you ever gotten dizzy looking at an optical illusion? That's a form of mental eyestrain.)

First, let's talk about the muscles that move your eyes. Each eye has six muscles controlling its movement, so that your eye can point up or down, left or right

(Figure 3). Those muscles get quite a daily workout – think about how many times your eyes have moved just reading this book!

The **medial rectus** and the **lateral rectus** are the muscles that control your eye's sideways movement. Whenever you look at something close, your eyes **converge**; that is, turn in toward your nose (Figure 4). If you look at anything that is extremely close (three feet away or less) for any length of time, as you do when reading, writing, or working on a VDT, the medial and lateral rectus muscles can become tired. If these muscles are weak to begin with, eye fatigue will occur faster. As you'll find out, eye muscles – just like any other muscle in your body – can be strengthened and toughened. The exercises at the end of this book will help.

Other candidates likely to be involved in eye-stress and VDT fatigue are the **ciliary** muscles (Figure 5). These are the muscles that focus the eye's lens. As your eye shifts to focus at various distances, the lens inside your eye is changing shape. Reading, for example, shapes the lens into something of a ball. Scanning the horizon flattens the lens. When the ciliary muscles relax, the lens naturally flattens out, automatically focusing for long-distance viewing. When you "tense up" these muscles for close work, they're likely to tire out fairly quickly. The same exercises that help the medial rectus and lateral rectus can also help the ciliary muscles.

Your ciliary muscles have an extraordinarily tough job, because the tiny lens inside the eye (continually balling up or flattening out as you change focus) is

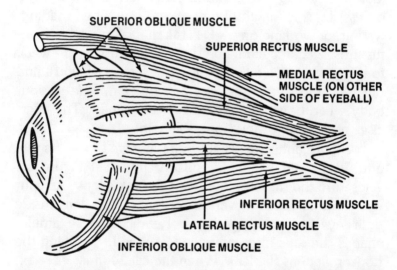

Figure 3. Six muscles move each eye. The medial and lateral rectus muscles are the ones that can become fatigued from extended viewing of a computer terminal.

becoming more rigid and less flexible with each passing day. As you age, your eyes will have an increasingly difficult time focusing for close work. Somewhere between the ages of 35 and 45, that lens will become quite rigid,

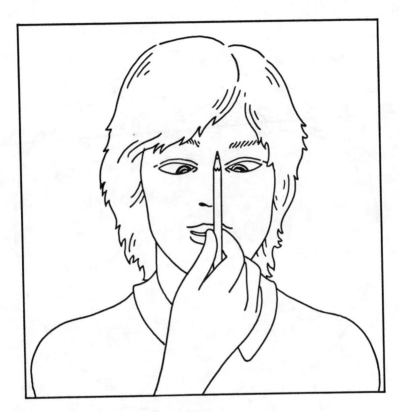

Figure 4. Looking at something close causes your eyes to converge, to turn in toward your nose. Doing this for any length of time can tire the muscles.

the muscles unable to do the work they did in your youth. The condition is known as **presbyopia**, and when it occurs, it's time for reading glasses or bifocals.

By the time you're 60, that tiny lens in your eye is

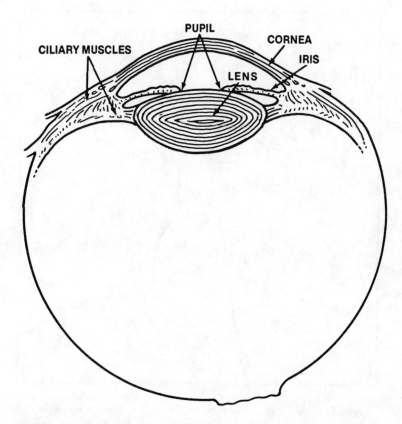

Figure 5. The ciliary muscles control the focusing of the lens inside the eye. These muscles must tense up to see objects that are close to you. They can become tired when the eyes are focused on a computer screen for a long period of time.

rock hard, and the ciliary muscles aren't having much effect on its shape. Ciliary-muscle exercises can't stop the aging and hardening process – but they *can* push the need for bifocals back a few years.

Did you know that the colored part of the eye, the **iris**), is almost all muscle? **Circular** muscles constrict the **pupil** (that black spot, actually a hole, in the center of the iris, and **radial** muscles dilate it. The pupil constricts or dilates in response to the amount of light striking the eye, so you can more easily adapt to dark or light conditions. (If you have a free moment, try standing in front of a bathroom mirror and switching the light off and on. You'll see how quickly and efficiently your eye muscles react.)

But changing illumination levels frequently and continually – by looking from a brightly lit document or page to a VDT, for example – can make these muscles ache. (It's like making your eyes do push-ups for eight hours straight!) Unfortunately, there aren't any exercises to help the matter – but there are things you can do to ease the strain. I'll be explaining these in detail farther along.

The last cause of eyestrain comes from the brain's efforts to decipher what is being seen. If you are reading along and suddenly what you are seeing is very blurred or obscured, your brain will say, "Hey, wait a minute, eye muscles, try to point both eyes at that line a little better. Ciliary muscle, let's get that word in better focus, and iris, make sure you are correcting for the light level and depth of focus. Let's even try squinting a little and furrowing the brow to see if that helps make things any clearer." So all of these muscles work a little harder on the blurred image. Your brain too has to work a little harder to figure out what it is seeing. If all these muscles and the brain have to work extra hard to figure out what is being seen, then pretty soon they are all tired out. Your eye movement muscles are tired; your ciliary muscles and iris are tired. Your eyelid muscles and the muscles around your eyes and forehead are tensed up. Your brain is tired. You are dealing with major eyestrain and headache.

SECTION 1
VDTs and Eyestrain

CHAPTER 1

You, Your Eyes, and VDT Fatigue

Now that we know what eyestrain is, let's consider why it is so often associated with video display use. VDT use involves concentrated close work with lots of opportunity for the display image to be somewhat blurry or difficult to read for one reason or another. VDT fatigue is the sum of many small factors. In order to prevent or at least limit VDT fatigue, we have to eliminate all of the small sources of discomfort so that we can stand to look at the VDT for a long period of time.

Let's discuss the individual problems that are sources of VDT fatigue.

Uncorrected Refractive Error

Uncorrected refractive error is a fancy term for certain kinds of eye problems that aren't being treated. If you need glasses but keep putting it off, or if your eyeglass prescription is out of date, then you're in the medical books. You have an uncorrected refractive error.

Frequently, patients who come to me for their regular eye examinations *think* they're seeing perfectly, when they're not seeing perfectly at all. In fact, many of them are seeing the world with fairly fuzzy or blurry vision! What they don't realize is that their vision has changed gradually over the years and they've subconsciously accustomed themselves to the changes. These people are amazed when I offer them a glimpse through a corrective lens!

People with visual problems, left untreated, are prime candidates for VDT fatigue. **Nearsightedness** (being able to see close objects clearly but not distant ones) often won't cause too much discomfort for an individual working with a VDT. But **farsightedness** is a VDT user's worst enemy. Farsightedness is being able to see distant objects more easily than close objects. Depending on its severity, farsightedness can make working on a VDT anything from mildly uncomfortable to agonizing.

Astigmatism is the name of yet another type of vision imperfection, an irregularity in the curvature of the front of the eye. Light rays entering an astigmatic eye do not meet at a single focal point. This results in a blurred or fuzzy image. Astigmatism is another source of VDT fatigue and, like farsightedness, it's easily cured by your friendly local optometrist.

There's one form of uncorrected refractive error that's particularly sneaky. That's a *small* degree of farsightedness. Slightly farsighted people can see distant objects clearly and they can also see close objects clearly, but not for long periods of time. For people with slight farsightedness, working in proximity to a VDT very quickly tires the ciliary muscles that focus the lens in the eye. Remember, the tiring of these muscles is one of the principal causes of eyestrain.

Before I go on, it's time to plug my profession. I recommend regular eye examinations for everyone, but they're particularly important for people who use VDTs regularly. I've seen enough damaged eyes, and have taken care of more than enough badly strained eyes, to emphatically recommend eye examinations once a year. I reiterate, *once a year*. Both the American Optometric Association and the National Institute of Occupational Safety and Health (NIOSH) recommend yearly eye examinations for VDT users. A prescription for glasses can often do wonders for VDT fatigue. Correction of even small refractive errors (a minor change in existing prescription glasses or a prescription for work glasses) can make a drastic difference.

Convergence and Focusing

Another cause of VDT fatigue is the eye's poor ability to converge and focus when looking at something close. Remember, when your eyes adjust to focus on a VDT, they turn inward. People who normally cannot cross their eyes easily are candidates for VDT fatigue. Poor ability to converge the eyes is often accompanied by poor focusing ability. Also, when working on a computer, you're often using a variety of focal points. Your eyes are shifting from the keyboard to the screen to your copy or some other information source. It's more eyework than just reading a book, for example.

I'm reminded of a patient of mine, Jenny, a good example of someone with convergence difficulty. Jenny is a mother of two who rejoined the work world after nine years of raising her children. Her new job entailed some four hours of VDT work each day. After only her second day on duty she was ready to throw in the towel. Her eyes ached and "grew sleepy" whenever she was using a computer. She went to an eye doctor, who told her that her eyes were fine. "No need for glasses," he assured her.

But the symptoms persisted and she came to me, on the verge of quitting her job. I checked her eyes, and sure enough, she wasn't nearsighted and she wasn't farsighted, nor did she have astigmatism. I could certainly understand how another eye doctor had missed the problem.

But I found that when I held a pencil about a yard away from her face and moved it toward her, the image would split in two about 18 inches from her eyes. Her medial rectus muscles (which control her ability to turn her eyes inward) were quite weak. As the pencil grew closer, her muscles would not maintain precise eye movement and her brain was actually "seeing" two pencils. In addition, after about ten round trips with the pencil, even her focusing ability tired – and she was ultimately seeing two *blurred* pencils!

Her treatment was threefold. First, I prescribed a pair of glasses that reduced her need to focus as intently. Then I gave her certain eye exercises to strengthen both her convergence muscles and her focusing muscles.(They're some of the same exercises you'll read about later.) Last, I gave her some very pertinent information, which has become the content of this book. Within two weeks, her eyes were much less tired by VDT work. Her productivity and efficiency had increased, and she was much happier at her job.

Easing the strain of VDT fatigue can do more than just increase your comfort. Like Jenny, you will increase your productivity as well (Figure 6). You'll find your workload – well, enjoyable. That's the difference this book can make!

Tension Level

Keeping yourself relaxed and as free as you can be from tension and worry helps minimize VDT fatigue. When you are excited or anxious or nervous, you have more difficulty focusing and converging your eyes on close objects. Your pupils are stimulated to dilate. The part of the nervous system that responds to fear, worry, or anxiety sends messages to all parts of the body to get ready to either fight or run away. This is known as the **sympathetic response** and comes from the sympathetic nervous system. This response stimulates your eyes to dilate, which makes it even harder for your eyes to converge and focus up close. If you have

Computer Eye-Stress

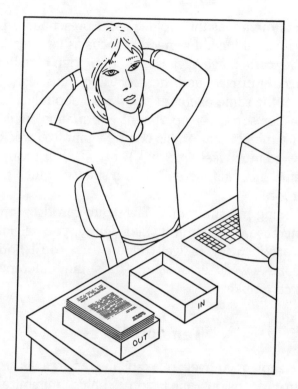

Figure 6. Easing the strain of VDT fatigue can increase your comfort and your productivity.

ever seen a cat or a dog that has just been frightened, you may have noticed that its eyes were widely dilated.

Well, when you are working under a lot of pressure, as so many computer users are (I've even heard it said that only air traffic controllers are more stressed than word processors working under a deadline, and even the air traffic controllers are using VDTs), your sympathetic nervous system is being stimulated. Your convergence and focusing muscles and your iris are being even more taxed to overcome the effects of the sympathetic nervous system. Learning to keep yourself relaxed will help a great deal in minimizing VDT fatigue.

Blinking

About a year ago a woman came to me who complained about having trouble reading because her eyes burned. But she was having trouble only while she was reading at work. She was a lawyer. If she read a novel, she didn't have any problem, but when reading a law brief, her eyes would burn and burn after about ten minutes. She kept putting eye drops in her eyes, which would help for a while, but pretty soon her eyes were burning again. This was very frustrating to her, because she loved her work and found all of her work-related reading stimulating and interesting. The glasses that she wore were the correct prescription, and the muscles of her eyes were well conditioned.

It turned out that whenever she read for her work, she would forget to blink. She would become so engrossed in what she was reading that she would subconsciously suppress the urge to blink, so her eyes would dry out and burn! As odd as it sounds, many people become so involved in what they are doing that they simply stare at their work. This is especially true for people working with computers, since this type of work demands extra concentration. The normal rate of blinking is about once every five seconds, but with intense staring, the rate can easily become once every minute or two. This will dry out your eyes and make them burn. For people who I suspect are having trouble blinking enough, I recommend that they "practice" blinking for a minute or so before they begin work. I want them to think about blinking so they will be a little more conscious of blinking correctly as they work with their VDT.

Along the same lines, people who don't have very good tear production or whose tears are not as thick and viscous as they should be can have similar problems. Their eyes can feel gritty and may burn when they stare at VDT terminals. For those who have naturally dry eyes, I recommend using an artificial tear occasionally as they work. There are several types that work well, such as Hypotears, Liquifilm Tears, and Tears Naturale. I do not recommend the type of eye drop that "gets the red out" for this kind of problem. In fact, I don't know any eye doctors who do recommend this type of drop, because it is too easy for your eyes to get addicted to it so that you have to use it every day.

CHAPTER 2

The Computer Work Station and VDT Fatigue

Lighting and Contrast

Until now, I have been discussing problems with the eyes and the muscles around the eyes. Now let's discuss lighting and illumination problems and the VDT screen itself. As you read this section, think about your own computer set-up – where the monitor sits, the lighting, and the characteristics of the VDT.

How did most computers arrive in offices? At some point, someone decided to go out and purchase one. Then someone brought it back to the office, moved the typewriter over, and plugged it in. Usually the computer has ended up in a place that was not designed to have a computer.

Most offices are twice as bright as they should be for looking at VDT screens. The eye has trouble adapting to both the bright room illumination and the lower light level

23

of the VDT screen. Also, the screen gets "washed out" by room illumination that is too bright. So, if you are working in a typical office, you will want to cut the lighting around the computer by half. If you think you work in a dimly lit dungeon of an office, it may be about right for a computer. If you work in a glassed-in patio, you should move indoors. Generally, what you may have to do is draw the shades and use lower-wattage bulbs or fewer fluorescent bulbs. Possibly a hood could be fitted over the computer that would decrease the illumination.

Let me remind you here that VDT fatigue is not usually due to one single factor. Most often it comes from having a number of little factors combine to cause eyestrain. Lowering the room illumination may not seem to be a big deal by itself. But it gets rid of one more factor that leads to VDT fatigue. Don't just be *aware* that your room is too bright; make sure that you are using the proper illumination level.

Like television sets, most VDTs have two knobs: one for adjusting the contrast, the other for adjusting the brightness. Many VDT users spend months working with their screens before they discover these controls. The brightness control adjusts the overall brightness of the screen, while the contrast control adjusts the brightness of the characters in relation to the screen background. The characters should be five to ten times brighter than the background. If the character contrast is not this high, the characters will be much harder to see. Of course, you are not going to try to measure the amount of contrast. Just find the brightness and contrast knobs and adjust the characters so that they are not too dim but not so bright that they flicker.

Quite a few of the VDTs available today have a negative contrast option. This lets you change from light letters on a dark background (positive contrast) to dark letters on a light background (negative contrast), more like the letters on a printed page. Unfortunately, the screens are more apt to flicker with negative contrast. Most users prefer the more normal positive contrast, but it is nice to use the negative contrast option occasionally to relieve boredom and to give your eyes a chance to look at something different.

Glare and Reflections

One of the biggest problems with VDTs is **glare**, which is light that's reflected off the glass surface (Figure 7). We all know how difficult it can be to read from books that have glossy pages. VDTs often have quite a bit of glare bouncing off the screen. I asked a friend of mine who is in real estate development and who uses a personal computer a great deal if his eyes bothered him. "Not particularly," he said, "but there are these five bright light reflections here on the screen that make it difficult to see." Sure enough, there were five very bright areas on the screen, so that he was always having to reposition his head and his eyes to see. His computer has been sitting at that spot in his office for a year and a half. He knows those glare spots annoy him and make him uncomfortable. He just hasn't taken the time to get rid of that glare.

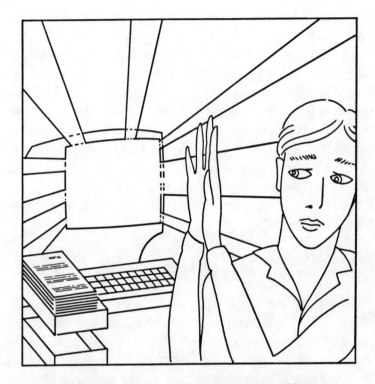

Figure 7. Glare, one of the biggest problems associated with VDTs, can be reduced with antiglare filters.

Remember that VDT fatigue can build up from several sources. Take the time to eliminate glare problems. This might involve moving a lamp or putting up some window shades. Maybe moving the computer to a different location will help. Antiglare filters are available that can be placed over the VDT screen. These can go a long way toward eliminating glare. Many of the newer and more expensive monitors are now being manufactured with the problem of screen glare taken into consideration. These monitors have antiglare coatings or antiglare screens built in that are quite effective. Don't put up with glare that obliterates your word processing or computer program. Take the time to locate the source of the glare and either eliminate it or screen it out.

Besides reflected glare from lights, other reflections in VDT screens are a problem. Bookcases or desks or people moving around in the background can be reflected in the VDT screen (Figure 8). What is so bad about reflections? Suppose there is a bookcase 20 feet behind you, and you can see its reflection in the VDT screen. While you work, your eyes are focused on the screen, less than two feet from you. Whenever you unconsciously focus your eyes on the reflection of the bookcase, they are actually focusing in direct proportion to the distance the bookcase – from eye to screen to bookcase. In other words, your eyes are constantly refocusing from a 2-foot to a 22-foot distance, back and forth, back and forth. This can lead to eyestrain. Positioning the VDT so that there are few objects in the background to cause reflections and using antiglare screens will minimize this problem.

The VDT Unit Itself

The quality of the VDT display has a great deal to do with the degree of VDT fatigue you will experience. The harder it is for you to make out the letters on the screen,

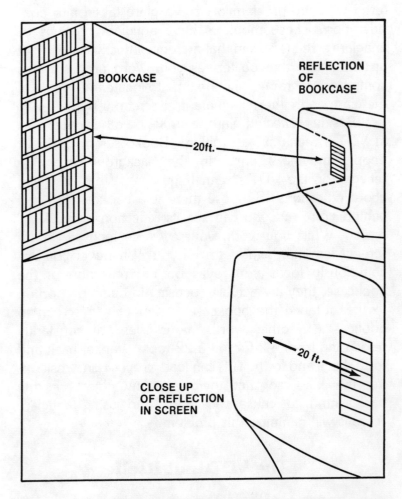

Figure 8. When you look from the text on the computer screen to a reflection on the screen, there is a drastic change in focus, because your eyes adjust their focus to include the object's distance from the screen.

the sooner fatigue will be upon you. Key factors here are the size and resolution of the letters and the style of type that is used.

One of the most common complaints of VDT users is that their screen flickers. This happens because the phosphor in the screen fades too quickly, the electron beam doesn't scan fast enough, or the monitor isn't getting the picture from the computer fast enough. Whatever the reason, you should avoid flickering screens. Try adjusting the brightness control to reduce your screen's flicker.

The last characteristic of computer monitors that matters to your eyes is the color used in the display. Certain colors are hard on your eyes, while others are more restful and easier to look at. Red or blue is probably the hardest on your eyes, while either green or amber is the easiest.

Part I of the two-part plan for reducing VDT fatigue will cover the features that distinguish a good computer monitor and talk about how best to design a computer work station to keep your VDT fatigue to a minimum.

CHAPTER 3

Other Factors and VDT Fatigue

Wearing Glasses with VDTs

If you wear glasses, then you have some extra problems to contend with while you are working with your computer. For some of you, these problems will be so minor that you won't pay them any attention. But for a lot of you, these problems with your glasses will be severe enough to be a central cause of your VDT fatigue. In this section, I will tell you how to wear your glasses comfortably.

But first, do you have to wear your glasses when you work with your computer? That depends on why you wear glasses in the first place. If you cannot read the monitor when you take your glasses off, then the answer to that question is pretty easy – yes, you have to wear your glasses. If you can read the monitor with your glasses off, then *maybe* you don't have to wear them.

If you have a low to moderate amount of near-sightedness, you can, without any difficulty, take your glasses off and work with the computer. In fact, you might even be more comfortable without your glasses. The problem you will have is seeing the clock on the wall with your glasses off. If you wear glasses for any reason other than small amounts of nearsightedness, then you should wear your glasses when you work with your computer – even if you can still see the monitor when you aren't wearing them. This will keep your eyes comfortable for long periods of time as you work. When you have your eyes examined, you should ask your doctor what your glasses correct for and when you should wear them. If you don't know whether you are nearsighted or if you wear glasses for another reason, call your doctor and ask.

If you are going to wear your glasses when you work, then you are going to want them to be comfortable. First and foremost, this means that you need a good-quality frame that is adjusted well to fit your face. It doesn't matter much whether the frame is plastic or metal, as long as it fits you. Otherwise, the glasses will hurt behind your ear or pinch your nose or slide down constantly. While this isn't eyestrain, it certainly is a bother that you don't need when you are concentrating in front of a computer.

Glasses can also be uncomfortable because they are too heavy. The usual reason for glasses being too heavy is that the lenses are made of glass. Using plastic lenses instead of glass will make the glasses much lighter and therefore much more comfortable. If you do use glass lenses, choose a small frame so that the glass lenses are not very big.

Naturally, you should keep your glasses clean and free from scratches. It is not easy to see computer monitors or anything else through smudged and scratched glasses. Plastic lenses scratch whenever they are cleaned without some type of liquid. The best way to clean glasses is to use soapy water or window cleaner on the lenses, and then wipe with a soft cloth. Another thing that will keep plastic lenses from scratching is the application of an antiscratch coating.

We already know glare and reflections from the computer screen are problems. So are glare, reflection, and ghost images from your glasses. Antireflective coatings that are put on lenses eliminate these reflections. A light tint in the lenses also helps. Most people wouldn't consider buying binoculars or camera lenses without making sure that the lenses are coated. The same should be true of the glasses that you wear all of the time and that you use with VDTs.

Without a doubt, the glasses wearers who have the most problems looking at computer screens are bifocal wearers. When you wear bifocals, you have to look through the bottom part of the lens in just the right way to see up close. You also have to position your head the correct distance from the screen for the bifocal. All too often this leaves your head and neck contorted as you try to see the monitor, and you wind up unable to see anything clearly or comfortably.

To handle this situation, you first need to make sure

that your glasses are adjusted absolutely perfectly. To allow you to look at computer screens comfortably, the bifocal will need to be a little bit higher than usual, so you don't have to tilt your head too far to see the screen (Figure 9). It is best if the bifocal is fairly wide, at least 28 millimeters.

If you are having trouble seeing the keyboard, the computer screen, and the copy you are working from clearly at the same time, then you may need trifocal lenses. These have an extra portion in the lens that is for intermediate distances (Figure 10). With this type of lens, it is possible to see clearly at just about any distance.

One type of trifocal is a lens that has no lines in it. In this lens, the power changes progressively from distant to close-up focus. The difficulty with the lens is that the intermediate and near zones are not very wide. Because of this, most people who use this lens need to move their head as they look at the screen. Since this constant shifting gets to be annoying, I usually don't recommend the lens without lines for computer users.

Instead, the trifocal segment for computer users should be extra deep and wide and should not be set too low in front of the eyes. A special trifocal is now available that is designed for working with computer terminals. It is called a CRT lens. The trifocal lines of the CRT lens go all the way across the lens, and the middle portion is extra deep. It is through the middle segment that you view the VDT. If you are having trouble with your current trifocal, this may be the lens for you.

Since computers pose special problems for people

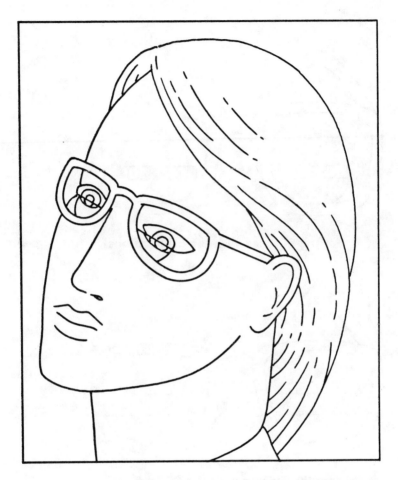

Figure 9. If the height of your bifocal is too low for computer work, your neck as well as your eyes will be uncomfortable. Talk to your doctor about how high your bifocal should be, and make sure your glasses are adjusted correctly.

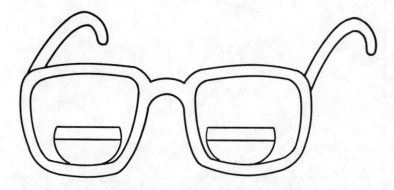

(a) Glasses with the usual trifocal.

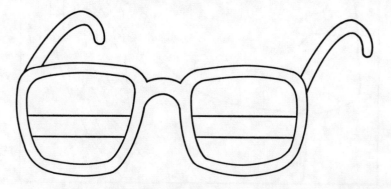

(b) Glasses with the CRT trifocal.

Figure 10. The CRT lens is a trifocal specifically made for working with computer terminals. The lens has an extra deep and wide intermediate section because this section is used the most when the wearer looks at a VDT.

who wear glasses, many wearers have one pair of glasses for general use and another just for looking at computer terminals. This solution lets you have glasses that you like for around the house or around town (such as the trifocal type that doesn't have any lines) without sacrificing clear vision or comfort when you work. The cost of a second pair of glasses may seem like a lot, but when you consider the added comfort and productivity, many times it's worth it.

Contact Lenses

For some people, wearing contact lenses can cause more problems with VDT screens than wearing glasses, while others have fewer problems with their contacts than with their glasses. It all depends on the fit of the contacts and the characteristics of the eyes.

There are two major types of contact lenses, hard and soft. Soft lenses are usually more comfortable than hard lenses when you first start wearing them. But some people cannot see as well with soft lenses and must use hard lenses. In either case, to wear contacts comfortably while working with a computer, you must have lenses that fit your eyes well. To make sure that you get a good fit, see an eye doctor who spends a great deal of time working with contact lenses. Also, make sure that your doctor has kept up with advances in contact lenses. The field changes so fast that it is easy for a doctor to get left behind if he or she doesn't work at staying current.

Computer Eye-Stress

When you first start wearing contact lenses, you will
have all of the problems associated with getting used to
contacts. These problems are worse for hard-lens wearers
than for soft-lens wearers. Your eyes are often a little red,
itchy, and teary; in general, they're not quite as comfortable as usual. During this adaptation time, it is especially
difficult to work with your computer, so it is a good idea
not to wear your contacts while using a VDT for the first
week. Let your eyes get used to the new sensations of
your contacts. Later, after you have adapted to the
lenses, you will find computer work more comfortable.

Even after you have adapted to wearing the lenses,
you will still have to keep several things in mind when
you are looking at the computer screen. The problems
that you can have with contact lenses and VDTs are pretty much the same whether you are wearing hard lenses,
soft lenses, lenses you sleep in, or lenses that correct
astigmatism.

First, it is so important to keep the lenses clean.
Deposits or residues on the lenses are probably the most
common cause of lens discomfort. You should follow
your doctor's advice to the letter to make sure that you
have clean lenses. If your lenses are irritating because
they aren't clean, you can bet that you will be think-
ing more about your lenses than your computer
monitor.

You have to blink when you wear contact lenses.
Blinking properly coats the lenses with tears and keeps
them wetted. It also pumps fresh tears under the lenses. If
you don't blink enough or don't blink your eyes completely

closed, the lenses will dry out and become uncomfortable. They may even pop out. A friend and patient of mine told me that the only time one of his soft lenses ever came out of his eye was when he was staring at his computer screen. He was staring and concentrating so hard that when he finally blinked, his dried-up soft lens popped out. Since he is now conscious of his need to blink when working with his computer, this hasn't happened again.

Computers are often in air-conditioned buildings. Sometimes, no matter how well or how frequently you blink, the air-conditioned environment will still dry out your eyes. When this happens, you might have to use some type of eye drop. Do not pick just any eye drop! Get your doctor to recommend one for your particular type of lens and your eyes.

Nearsightedness is by far the most common reason for wearing contacts. When nearsighted people wear contacts, they have to converge their eyes more than they do when they look through their glasses. This is because the lenses sit right on their eyes rather than sitting half an inch or so away as glasses do. For the same reason, the eyes must also focus a little more with contacts than with glasses. This means that nearsighted contact-lens wearers often need to strengthen their eye muscles when they are using computer monitors. New contact-lens wearers and people in their late thirties or early forties notice this problem the most. The best treatment is doing the eye exercises for reducing VDT fatigue presented at the end of this book.

The fact that a person is over 40 does not mean that he or she can't wear contacts and work with a computer. It does mean that computer work will probably be a little more difficult. There are bifocal hard lenses, bifocal soft lenses, and something called **monovision**. Monovision means wearing one contact lens for distance in one eye and at the same time wearing a contact lens for near vision in the other eye. All of these methods work for seeing both at a distance and close up with contact lenses. But how well they work depends on your own individual eyes and the skill of your doctor in fitting the lenses. Probably the easiest way to wear contacts when you are over 40 is to wear the lenses for distance and put on a pair of reading glasses when you sit down in front of the computer.

Contact-lens wearers can have problems while looking at VDT screens that others don't have. To keep from being hampered by your lenses, you will have to keep them clean, blink right, strengthen your eye muscles, and make sure that you have the correct fit for your eyes. Regular check-ups to make sure the lenses are continuing to fit correctly will ensure that your lenses stay comfortable.

Children and VDT Viewing

Children are taking to computers like fleas to a dog. They can't get enough. If they can't write programs for computers yet, then they can at least play games on them. They love having direct control over something.

Schools are teaching more and more computer classes. The school district in my area begins teaching children the computer keyboard in kindergarten. Kids at all grade levels are enjoying computers. They are staying after school on their own to use the computer. They are plunking down quarters in video arcades. And they are begging Mom and Dad to buy a home computer.

When television first came into the home, parents wondered about its effect on their children's eyes. To prevent or relieve eyestrain, they could always tell their kids to sit farther away. Not so with the computer screen. Children are going to have their eyes just a foot away from it (Figure 11). What can this do to their eyes?

Although it has not been proven, but many scientists and eye doctors think that too much close work for children causes nearsightedness. Their theory is that when the eye is focused on close objects too much, the eyeball becomes stretched. The eyeball then becomes too long, causing nearsightedness. To keep this from happening, many eye doctors prescribe eye glasses that will reduce the amount of focusing that a child has to do. This will then keep the eye from stretching too much and possibly causing nearsightedness.

Color Vision Deficiencies

About 8 percent of males are color defective. A much smaller number of females are color defective, less than 0.5 percent. I don't like to use the term "color blind," because these people do see color. However, they

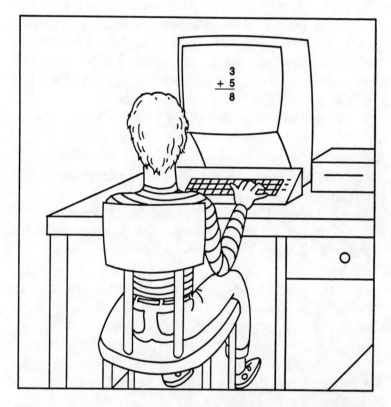

Figure 11. With children sitting just a foot away from VDT screens,many scientists and eye doctors worry that children may become nearsighted.

see colors slightly differently than everyone else, so they have difficulty discriminating among certain shades of color that people with normal color vision can easily tell apart.

A color that color-defective individuals commonly have trouble identifying is green, a color frequently used for VDT screens. I have been asked if this presents a problem for color defective VDT users. The answer is that it does *not* present a problem. Color-defective individuals may not be able to tell that they are looking at a green screen; they may think that it is white or gray or some other color. However, they will be able to see the letters on the screen as well as anyone else. If their eyes bother them, it is not because they are color defective. Some other cause of VDT fatigue, such as glare or poor focusing ability, is the source of their problems.

Radiation Dangers?

Way back when VDT users started noticing that their eyes ached, the first possible cause that occurred to them was "radiation" coming from the VDT. In fact, a number of patients have mentioned to me their fear that their eyes are being damaged by radiation from VDTs. One patient in particular comes to mind. He began to notice that if he used his green VDT screen for several hours, when he turned away from the screen, objects around the room glowed pink for several minutes. He felt sure that this was a sign that his eyes were being permanently damaged by radiation. Well, I managed to set his mind at rest, and I would like to do away with any similar fears you may have also. It is extremely unlikely that there is any sort of radiation hazard at all from VDTs. Every scientific study that has tried to find some type of dangerous radiation coming from VDTs has failed. The pink glow that my patient was noticing is a normal afterimage that comes from staring at a green VDT screen for a long time. You don't need a computer monitor to have this happen; staring at a green piece of paper for a long time can produce the same effect.

Let me just mention the types of radiation that could possibly come from VDTs: ultraviolet (UV) light, infrared radiation (IR), and X rays. A person out of doors is getting ten thousand times more UV from sunlight than he does in front of a VDT. Sunlight exposes a person to 100 to 1000 times more IR than a VDT screen. So neither ultraviolet nor infrared radiation is a problem. What about X rays? The screens made in the United States are all carefully manufactured to absorb X rays. So none escape to affect the user.

It is important that researchers keep measuring and testing the radiation levels of VDT screens to make sure that there never is a radiation danger from them. For now, however, the scare claims that VDTs cause cataracts or birth defects or miscarriages or skin rashes simply are not true.

SECTION 2

Two-Part Plan for Reducing VDT Fatigue

CHAPTER 4

Part I: The VDT
and the Work Station

The two-part plan outlined here puts together everything that I have described in this book into an effective, easy-to-do program for reducing VDT fatigue. Of course, the places where you find VDTs and the uses to which they are put are legion. It would be impossible to describe how every user should change his or her work environment to suit the computer. So I will describe the ideal conditions for the VDT user who spends three or more hours a day looking at a computer terminal. Part I will list the features to look for if you are buying a computer terminal and will describe the ideal work station and lighting conditions. Part II will tell you what to do to help your eyes stand up to the strain of using a computer terminal.

The VDT

As I have already said, the monitor itself and where it is placed will make a difference in how much strain your eyes endure. Many of you will think that you have no control over these factors. You or your company probably already own the computer. There may be some good reason why the computer has to go in this particular room under these particular lighting conditions that are not ideal. But if reducing VDT fatigue is important to you, think about what you can do to make your situation more like the ideal. If your VDT display is terrible, you don't have to buy a new computer. Good, reasonably priced (about $150) monitors can be individually purchased and added on to most computers. Tilting the screen differently or attaching an antiglare filter may be all that you can do to change your work station, but even this simple change may reduce the strain on your eyes. If you are about to purchase a computer for your home or office, then you will have a chance to put all of the recommendations in this book into effect.

VDTs that have poor display characteristics are a cause of VDT fatigue. The important characteristics are the legibility of the characters, the amount of screen flicker, and the color of the display.

Several factors determine the legibility of the characters. The size of the standard character is important. Obviously, a five-inch diagonal screen is going to need smaller letter sizes than a larger screen to display as much information. The style of type also makes a difference.

You probably want one that looks like standard English letters and not like hieroglyphics. The letters should seem solid and have good resolution. If there is too much space between the dots that make up each letter, then the letters will be difficult to read.

When you look at the screen, you should notice very little flicker, if any. If the screen seems to be flickering too much, try turning down the brightness. This will often cut down on the flicker that you see.

Many computers now offer the option of having either a monochrome (one-color) or a multiple-color VDT. Green or amber monochrome screens are easier on your eyes than black and white or any other color. Multiple colors can be useful for displaying graphs, highlighting important points, working with computer animation, and so on. But when you need to get down to work and write programs, do word processing, or perform any other task that means you are going to stare at the screen for a period of time, use just one color. Again, the best color to use is either green or amber.

Another point to consider about color monitors is that the least expensive of them have very poor resolution for letters and numbers. The most expensive red-green-blue (RGB) monitors work much better. If you have to work with a lot of text on the screen but can only afford an inexpensive color monitor, you and your eyes will be much better off if you purchase an even less expensive monochrome monitor.

Most VDTs have controls for adjusting brightness and contrast. The brightness of the whole screen should be three to four times the overall room illumination, and the characters on the screen should be five to ten times brighter than the screen background.

Many of the newer monitors are already equipped with antiglare coatings or screens. This is a super feature. When you compare a screen that has a good filter to one that doesn't, it is obvious that the one with the filter is much easier on your eyes. It is possible to buy separate add-on filters from computer stores. If the VDT you have doesn't have an antiglare filter, I urge you to get one.

Another thing that can help reduce glare is changing the way the VDT is tilted or swiveled. Some VDTs are fully adjustable. For those that are not, try improvising with books or pads to improve the tilt of the monitor. Tilting and swiveling stands are also available for computer monitors.

In order to detect and get rid of the glare that is reflected in the screen, sit in front of the screen with the computer off. Whatever you can see in the screen now is going to be there in the way when you are using the computer. Draw shades to get rid of window light. Move lamps, shield lamps, close doors, and do whatever else you can do to get rid of bright, reflecting lights. If you have trouble telling where a bright light is coming from, move a book or piece of paper around in front of the screen and observe when the glare is blocked out.

It is a good idea not to wear a light-colored top when you work with the computer. Light reflecting from your white shirt might make you a glare source.

The overall room illumination should be about half

what you usually find in offices. The desired level is 30 to 50 footcandles and is about equivalent to the light given off by a 60-watt bulb in a small room. It is ideal if the computer can have its own special room where the illumination can be adjusted. Then a small adjustable lamp can be used to light up whatever document or paperwork you might be using.

The Work Station

It is important that the video display and keyboard be placed so they can be viewed easily, without causing undue postural strain to either your neck or your back. In fact, in addition to eyestrain, body aches and pains are a common complaint of VDT users. Designing a work station that will allow the user to sit and work comfortably will go far toward relieving eye and posture strain (Figure 12). The more components of the work station that are individually adjustable – screen height, chair height, and so on – the better.

- The VDT screen should be 15° below the user's horizontal line of sight. The viewing distance from the user's eyes to the screen should be about 50 centimeters, or 18 inches.

- If you are working from hard copy (that's computerese for pieces of paper), this would ideally be placed at the same height and distance as the VDT screen. This will allow for a minimum of head movement and change of focus as you

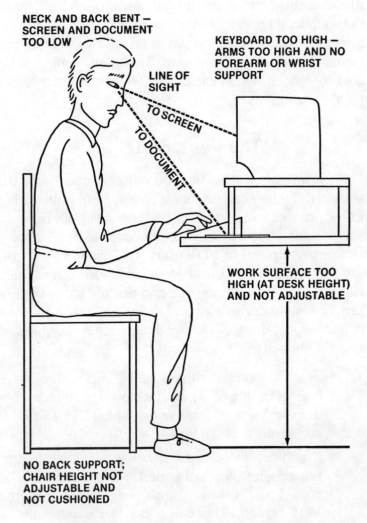

Figure 12a. A poorly designed work station.

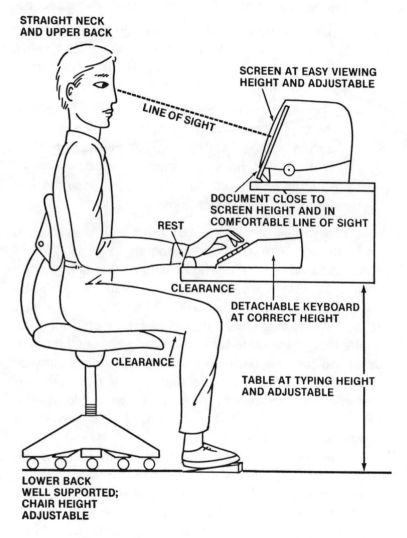

STRAIGHT NECK AND UPPER BACK

SCREEN AT EASY VIEWING HEIGHT AND ADJUSTABLE

LINE OF SIGHT

DOCUMENT CLOSE TO SCREEN HEIGHT AND IN COMFORTABLE LINE OF SIGHT

REST

CLEARANCE

DETACHABLE KEYBOARD AT CORRECT HEIGHT

CLEARANCE

TABLE AT TYPING HEIGHT AND ADJUSTABLE

LOWER BACK WELL SUPPORTED; CHAIR HEIGHT ADJUSTABLE

Figure 12b. A well-designed work station.

look from the VDT screen to the hard copy.

- The keyboard should be about 30 inches from the floor, so that the upper arms hang vertically while the forearms angle down slightly from horizontal. A palm rest can be added to support the wrists.

- The chair should be of adjustable height so that the thighs can be horizontal. It should be well supported with either four legs or five casters. The chair should have a backrest, including lumbar support. A footrest can be used, or else the feet should be flat on the floor.

You should also pay attention to your overall work environment. Are you a nonsmoker in a roomful of smokers? Perhaps it's not VDT fatigue that is bothering your eyes; maybe it's just your office mate's cigarette. Is the room temperature comfortable? Or do you work in an office building that cranks up the heat so high during the winter that you want to wear shorts and has you bundling up in the summer because the air conditioner's thermostat seems to have only one setting – for 62°? Do you wish that the secretary in the other room would at least turn the radio to a better station, if not turn if off altogether?

The quality of your overall work environment is going to affect your general performance and state of mind. Overall quality of the work environment includes how you feel about your job. Does your job offer you enough stimulation, responsibility, creativity, security, pay? Most jobs that have computers associated with them are jobs that exert a fair amount of pressure on the employees. As I have said before, the more stressed you are for any reason, the more likely it is that your eyes are going to be fatigued by looking at a computer terminal. Because of this, you should work toward making your overall work station and work environment as comfortable as possible. You might be surprised to discover that the secretary in the next room doesn't mind turning her radio down when she discovers that it annoys you.

CHAPTER 5

Part II: You and Your Eyes

If you have not done so recently, pick up the telephone, call an optometrist, and make an appointment to have your eyes examined. Find out if you have any special vision problems that need correcting. I recommend eye examinations every year for VDT users – every six months if you wear contact lenses.

Learn to relax! Take rest breaks. Give your eyes, your mind, and your body regular breaks from using the computer. As you work, occasionally look up and focus across the room or out the window. If you are using the VDT a moderate amount (looking at the monitor less than 50 percent of the time), then you should take a 15-minute break every two hours. You don't have to take a coffee break, but you should do something other than computer work during that time.

Relaxation therapy is a very good thing to do occasionally during a rest break. This will help remove tenseness from your body, make your eyes feel more relaxed, and actually give you more energy to continue

Computer Eye-Stress

your work. Doing this two to three times a day will give you the most benefit.

This is a good way to relax:

a. Find a quiet spot where you can sit or lie comfortably. Close your eyes. If you are sitting, rest your face in the palms of your hands.

b. Take several deep breaths to begin. Then breathe normally.

c. Start with the muscles around your eyes. Tell yourself that tension is draining from them and that those muscles are becoming relaxed. Next tell yourself that your head and neck muscles are becoming relaxed. Work your way down your body, relaxing the muscles in your shoulders and back, arms, stomach, hips and thighs, calves and feet. Work your way back up your body, directing your thoughts to further relax all of your muscles, ending where you started – with your eyes.

d. Imagine yourself in peaceful, pleasant surroundings. Imagine that you are relaxed and content.

e. Finally, imagine yourself getting up from your peaceful surroundings and doing some energetic activity that you enjoy. Think of the feeling of abundant energy and enthusiasm that you have as you do this activity.

f. Open your eyes and feel how refreshed you are. You can then continue with your computer work.

Eye Muscle Exercises

The following exercises are recommended for everyone. They will help strengthen the muscles that turn the eye in and out and the muscles that help focus the lens in the eye. They will benefit those who notice letters and words splitting in two or blurring, those who find that it takes several seconds to refocus their eyes after looking at a VDT, and those in their late 30s or early 40s who do not use reading glasses. The great thing is that they are easy to do and don't take much time.

Take note. If you don't do the exercises – they can't work. In other words, you have to do the exercises for five to ten minutes a day for at least two weeks before you notice any benefit. If you don't do the exercises, you won't notice any benefit. A way to make sure you do them is to incorporate them in your daily routine. Those of you who rise early enough for a leisurely breakfast should do them before or after that meal. The rest of us late risers will have to do them at lunch. I think that the most disagreeable time to do the exercises is at night when you are already tired from work, but the important thing is to do them. They will help keep your eye muscles from getting tired, so you will suffer less eye fatigue. One nice thing is that after three weeks to a month, your eye muscles will be strong enough to allow you to do the exercises somewhat less regularly.

When you do the exercises, you should expect them to be difficult at first, even to the point of making your eyes ache as you do them. These exercises are like any others: when you are doing the exercises your muscles will hurt, but they will make your muscles stronger in the long run.

Everyone will begin these exercises at his or her own level of ability. If your eye muscles are already in good shape, then you will be able to proceed quickly through the exercises and on to a maintenance program. If your muscles are a bit sluggish, it might take five to six weeks before you go on a maintenance program. If you are never able to do Exercise 1, then you should see an eye doctor for individualized attention.

The program is set up in blocks of exercises. Start with Block 1. When you have mastered the exercise in Block 1, continue on to Block 2, and so forth. If you wear glasses for any reason (even if they are only for distance), wear them while you do the exercises.

Block 1

Block 1 consists of Exercise 1 only – beads and string. (The description of the exercises begins on page 63.) The purpose of this exercise is to enable both eyes to see the same object at the same time, which you must be able to do to complete the program. Work with this exercise for 10 to 15 minutes a day. As soon as you can easily do the exercise, move on to Block 2. This may be after only one exercise session, or it may be after several. If you cannot do this exercise after a two-week period, then you will have difficulty doing the rest of the exercises and you should see your eye doctor about this problem.

Block 2

- Begin Block 2 with Exercise 2 and do two sets of 20 repetitions.
- Repeat this the next day.
- On the following day, add one set of 20 repetitions of Exercise 3.
- Repeat this for the next one to four days, depending on how hard the exercises seem to you. If they seem difficult and your eyes are really straining, do these exercises all four days. If they seem easy, move on to Block 3.

Block 3

In Block 3, continue with one set each of Exercises 2 and 3, but begin working with Exercise 4a. This exercise introduces the eccentric circles, which are challenging but fun. As with the beads and string exercises, some of you will be able to do this exercise very quickly, while most of you will take several sessions before you can do 4a easily. As soon as 4a is easy for you, move on to Block 4.

Block 4

- Do one set of Exercise 2 and one set of Exercise 4b the first day.
- The next day, do one set of Exercise 3 and one set of Exercise 4c.

- The next two days, do one set each of Exercises 4b, 4c, and 4d.
- To finish this block of exercises, do two sets each of Exercises 4b, 4c, and 4d for at least three days. When these exercises seem easy to you, move to Block 5.

Block 5

These are your maintenance exercises. You should do at least two sets of any exercise (from 2 through 4d) each week. Of course, more is better. You can do the exercises as often as you like. Maintenance exercises can easily be done during rest breaks from your computer work or during television commercials.

Exercise 1 – Beads and String

Purpose: To get both eyes to see the same object at the same time.

Procedure

You will need a string about seven feet long and two beads or buttons. Tie one end of the string to a door handle and place both beads on the string. Sit with the other end of the string pulled up to your nose (Figure 13). Position one bead about one-third of the way from the door handle and the other about one-third of the way from your nose. Look at the first bead. You may see one of three things (Figure 14). Figure 14c shows what you are supposed to see. If you see 14a, only your right eye is seeing and your left eye is suppressed. If you see 14b, only your left eye is seeing and your right eye is suppressed. In order to see 14c, try blinking your eyes rapidly, or shake the string. If this doesn't work, move the beads to different locations until you do see the beads and string as in Figure 14c.

Once you can see 14c, look at the far bead. You should see the pattern shown in Figure 14d. Again, work at seeing this. Once you have seen both 14c and 14d, reposition the beads and practice using both eyes at the same time at a number of points along the string. It may take only ten minutes, or it may take several practice sessions to do this.

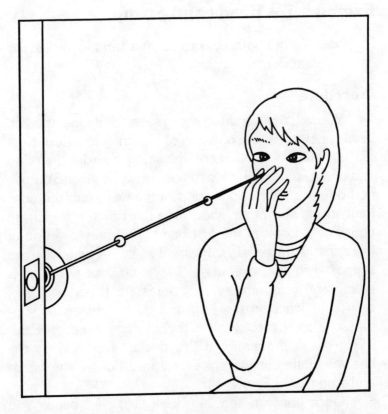

Figure 13. Use a string approximately seven feet in length and two beads or buttons to do Exercise 1.

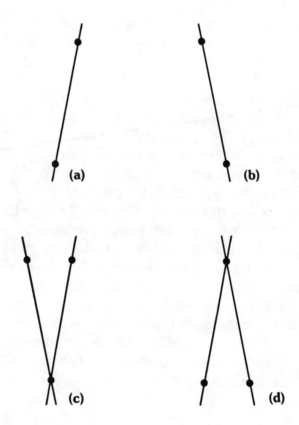

Figure 14. The beads and string exercises. (a) Appearance of beads and string if only the right eye is seeing; (b) Appearance of beads and string if only the left eye is seeing; (c) Beads and string as they should appear when you focus both eyes on the near bead; (d) Beads and string as they should appear when you focus both eyes on the far bead.

Exercise 2 – Pencil Push-Ups

Purpose: To improve your convergence and focusing abilities. This exercise will help both.

Procedure

Keep both eyes open for this exercise. Hold a pencil or pen about 20 inches in front of you. Look at the tip of the pencil. Bring the pencil toward you slowly and smoothly, keeping the tip clear. When the tip blurs, push the tip away from you until it is again 20 inches away. Concentrate on keeping the tip clear for as long as you can. Repeat this exercise ten times (Figure 15). On the eleventh repetition, keep bringing the pencil toward your nose even after the tip has blurred. Now try to keep the tip single for as long as you can. When the tip of the pencil splits in two or when the pencil gets to your nose, push the pencil away to the original starting position. Continue with this exercise in this manner for another ten repetitions to complete one set. The goal of this exercise is to move the point at which the pencil tip blurs and the point where it breaks in two closer and closer to you.

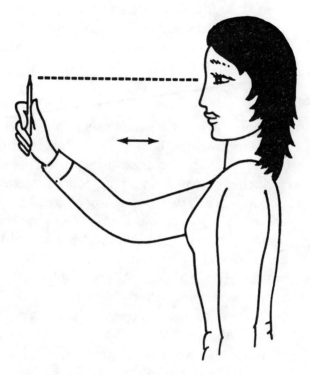

Figure 15. Pencil push-ups will help improve both convergence and focusing abilities.

Exercise 3 – Focusing Jumps

Purpose: To increase your ability to change from distant to close focus quickly and easily. This is an excellent exercise for strengthening your ciliary muscles and the muscles that converge and diverge your eyes.

Procedure

Again you will need a pencil or a pen for this exercise. Find an object that is at least 20 feet away from where you are sitting, and that has some visual detail, such as a clock on the wall. Hold the pencil tip directly in front of you and in line with the distant object. The pencil tip should be so close to you that it is almost, but not quite, at the blur point. First, look at the pencil tip. It should be crisp and clear. If it is not, move the pencil away from you until it is clear. As you are looking at the pencil tip, notice that the distant object is doubled (Figure 16). Then look at the distant object. When it is clear and sharp, notice that there are two pencils.

To perform this exercise, change your focus from the pencil tip to the distant object and back again to the pencil tip. This is one complete cycle. It is crucial to the success of this exercise that you change focus only when first, the object you are looking at is clear, and second, the other object appears doubled. This exercise should be done for 20 cycles to make up one set. The goal of this exercise is to increase the speed with which you can do the 20 cycles. But don't get sloppy as you get faster;

always make sure the two criteria are satisfied before you change focus.

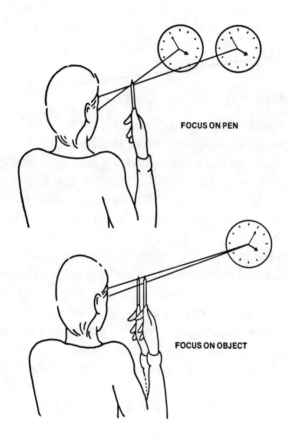

FOCUS ON PEN

FOCUS ON OBJECT

Figure 16. When doing focusing jumps, make sure the object that you are looking at is clear and the other object is seen as though it is split in two.

Exercise 4 – Eccentric Circles

Purpose: This is the most helpful exercise in this book but
also the most difficult. The procedures using eccentric circles work on convergence, diver-
gence, and focusing. They also help both eyes
to fixate accurately, and they increase your
depth perception.

Procedure A

You will need a pair of eccentric circle cards. Mount
the eccentric circle diagrams at the back of this book on
two cards, or make your own using a quarter and a dime
as templates to trace around. The eccentric circles should
look exactly like Figure 17. Hold the cards together in
one hand about 15 inches in front of you. The inner
circles should be on the inside; make sure that one card is
not held higher than the other. In the other hand, hold a
pencil halfway between the cards and your eyes. As you
look at the pencil, you will see the cards in the
background in one of two ways. You will see either three
cards or four (Figure 18). You want to see three cards. If
you see four, hold the pencil still and bring the cards
closer to you until the two inside cards merge into one.
When you see three cards, you will want to try to keep
that feeling in your eyes so that you can take the pencil
away and still see three.

The cards will probably appear blurry. I cannot ex-
plain how to see the center card image as being clear, but
as you look at the cards and concentrate on making them

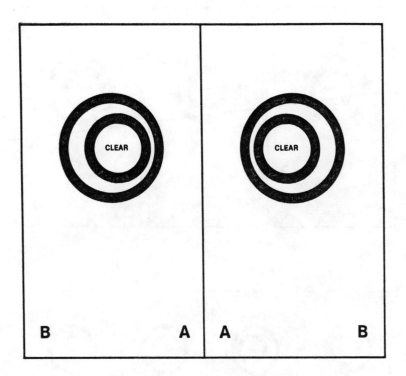

Figure 17. Two eccentric circle cards.

clear, they will eventually become so. The center card image should look different from the other two. In fact, the circles should look three-dimensional, as if you are looking into a bucket. When you can make the center card clear and three-dimensional, you are ready for the other exercises with the cards.

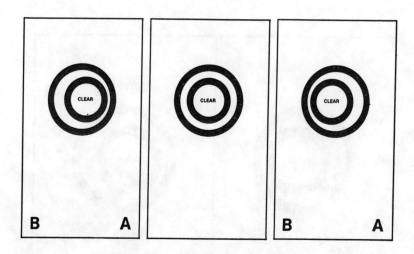

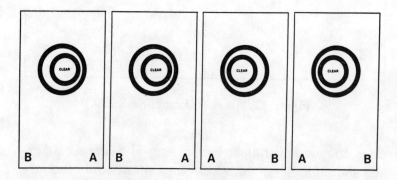

Figure 18. Using procedure A you want to see three cards as shown above. If you see four cards as shown in the second set of cards, hold the pencil still and bring the cards closer to you until the two inside cards merge into one.

Procedure B

Hold the cards about 15 inches in front of you. Cross your eyes so that you see three cards and the center one is clear and three-dimensional. Using both hands, slowly move the cards apart. Try to continue seeing the center card as clear and three-dimensional. At some point it will probably become blurry. Keep slowly pulling them apart until the center card image splits into two. Then push the cards back together, maintaining your clear view of the center card. Do this for two minutes. Keep trying to move the cards farther apart before the image blurs and splits into two.

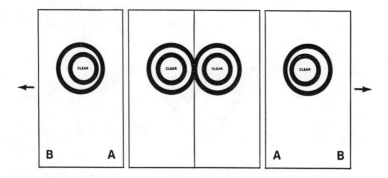

Figure 19. When you begin procedure B, the cards should appear as in the top portion of Figure 18. If you keep pulling the cards apart, you will end up with the view shown in the bottom portion of Figure 18.

Procedure C

This time, instead of moving the cards apart, bring them toward you. Again, try to bring the cards closer and closer to you before they blur and split in two (Figure 20). Then push them back away from you. Repeat this for two minutes.

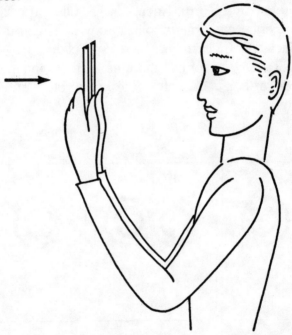

Figure 20. The pair of cards should appear to be double.

Procedure D

Hold the cards 15 inches away and cross your eyes so that the center image is clear and three-dimensional. Then look away to a distant object. After that object is clear, look back at the cards and quickly try to make the center image clear and three-dimensional. Then look back at the distant object. Repeat this for two minutes. The goal is to have the center image quickly snap clear and three-dimensional.

Conclusion

The advice, recommendations, and exercises in this book will help you work with computer terminals better. Remember that VDT fatigue usually comes from a combination of many small problems. The closer you come to working under the ideal conditions, the better for your eyes. Certainly many situations will be impossible to change. I don't expect that, for example, airports will start cutting down on the terminal lights overnight so that the ticket agents have an easier time of it, but making bosses and planners aware of these ideal conditions is important. Point out that the closer your work environment is to these ideal conditions, the more productive you will be. You might possibly start to see changes in your work place that will make the VDT user's eyes more comfortable.

Doing what you can for your eyes will make you more productive and will make your relationship with your computer all the better.

Index

Computer Eye-Stress

ciliary muscles, 7-11, 17
circular muscles, 11
lateral rectus, 7
medial rectus, 7, 18
radial muscles, 11
see also Presbyopia
Eyeglasses, 31-37
bifocals, 33-34
cleaning, 33
CRT lens, 34
frame adjustment, 32
ghost images, 33
glare, 33
multiple pairs, 37
reflections, 33
scratches, 33
trifocal lenses, 33-34
wearing of, 31-32
weight, 32-33
Eyestrain, 6-12
causes, 6
mental eyestrain, 11-12
see also VDT fatigue

Focusing, 17-19

Glare; *see* VDT glare reduction

Headaches, 1, 12

Iris, 11

Lens, 7-1
changes with age, 8-11

Monitor; *see* VDT
Muscles; *see* Eye muscles

Presbyopia, 8-11
Pupil, 11

Radiation, 43-44
infrared radiation (IR), 44
ultraviolet (UV) light, 44
X rays, 44
Relaxation therapy, 57-58
Room illumination, 50-51

Television, 5-6
Trifocal lenses, 34
CRT lens, 34

Uncorrected refractive error, 15-17
astigmatism, 16
farsightedness, 16
nearsightedness, 16
slight farsightedness, 17

VDT, 2-3
brightness adjusting, 24, 49-50
character legibility, 48-49
contrast adjusting, 24, 49-50
definition, 4-6
display colors, 28, 49
flickering, 28, 49
glare; *see* VDT glare reduction
phosphor, 5-6
quality and VDT
fatigue, 27-28, 48
radiation hazards; *see* Radiation
raster structure, 5
red-green-blue (RGB)
monitors, 49
resolution, 49
VDT fatigue, 3-4, 15-23

About the Author

Dr. Hutchinson received his Bachelor of Arts degree from the University of California at Los Angeles and his Doctor of Optometry degree from the University of California at Berkeley. His professional activities include membership in the San Diego County Optometric Society, the California Optometric Association, and the American Optometric Association. An area of special interest is the effect of video display terminals on the vision of computer users. His practice also includes prescription of contact lenses and contact lens research. He is a member of the American Optometric Association's section on contact lenses. Dr. Hutchinson also has extensive experience in screening school children for vision problems.

Eccentric Circles
for Your Cards

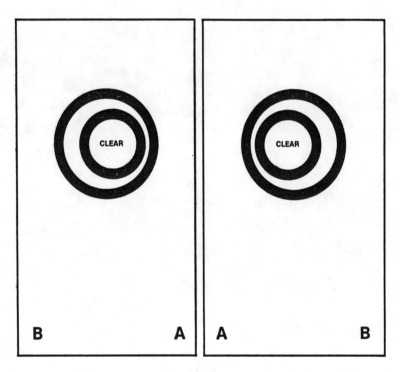

Cut out these two cards and mount them separately on card stock or cardboard. For an explanation of the use of the eccentric circle cards see page 70.

"A must for all computer users. This book is outstanding in helping to solve the problems computer users have with their eyes."

Gerald Easton, O.D.,
President of The American Optometric Association,
(1985–86)

After a long session at your computer screen, are you bothered by any of these symptoms:
   headache?
   itching eyes?
   blurred vision?
   burning eyes?
   double vision?

Over 75 percent of computer users report some form of visual discomfort while using a terminal.

In his book, California optometrist R. Anthony Hutchinson offers a two-part program of relief. In the first, he shows you how to situate yourself and your VDT to minimize the problem. In the second, he offers eye exercises to strengthen your eye muscles and enable them to deal better with the strains of computer use. There are sections for those who wear eyeglasses and contact lenses and a special section about children and VDT viewing.

DR. HUTCHINSON received his Doctor of Optometry degree from the University of California at Berkeley. He practices in San Diego.

Cover Design by Bob Silverman
Health/Computers/Business

ISBN   0-87131-457-6   > > $4.95

FPT   0481-140